HOW TO IMPROVE THE BRAIN

"Unleash Your Brain's Potentials"

William T. Pruitt

Disclaimer

The information contained in this book is not intended to be a substitute for professional medical advice, diagnosis, or treatment. Always seek the advice of your physician or other qualified healthcare provider with any questions you may have regarding a medical condition.

Information provided in this book is based on research and is intended for educational purposes only

The author and publisher of this book are not responsible for any errors or omissions, or for any actions taken based on the information contained in this book. The author and publisher shall have no liability or responsibility to any person or entity with respect to any loss or damage caused, or alleged to be caused, directly or indirectly, by the information contained in this book.

By using the information contained in this book, you acknowledge and agree that you have read and understand this disclaimer and that you release the author and publisher from any liability.

Table of Content

Introduction

Unleash Your Brain's Potential

First Chapter

The Human Brain

Second Chapter

Brain Health Nutrition

Third Chapter

Physical Activity and Brain Power

Fourth Chapter

Cognitive Training and Mental Stimulation

Fifth Chapter

Sleep Quality for Cognitive Enhancement

Sixth Chapter

Stress Reduction and Emotional Well-Being

Seventh Chapter

Social Relationships and Brain Health

Eight Chapter

Nootropics and Brain Enhancement Supplements

Ninth Chapter

"The Journey to a Better Brain."

<u>Introduction</u>

Unleash Your Brain's Potential

The human brain is one of the most amazing and complicated organs known to man. It is the hub of our ideas, emotions, creativity, and memories, as well as the command-and-control center for all physical functions. Despite this, many of us are only scratching the surface of what our minds are capable of.

Throughout history, scientists, scholars, and individuals have been fascinated by the quest to unleash the full potential of the human brain. From ancient philosophers delving into the depths of human cognition to modern neuroscientists tracing the intricate networks of the brain, our understanding of this amazing organ has grown dramatically.

There has been a rise in interest in improving brain health and cognitive performance in recent years. People are actively exploring ways to optimize their brainpower, whether it's to sharpen memory, boost creativity, improve focus, or simply preserve a healthy brain as we age.

This book, "How to Improve the Brain," will accompany you on a journey of self-discovery, self-improvement, and unlocking the potential of your brain. It will look at the various facets of brain health and cognitive enhancement, drawing on the most recent scientific research as well as practical tactics that may be easily implemented in your daily life.

Our voyage will take us through the brain's inner workings, uncovering the wonders of its structure and function. We'll look at nutrition, exercise, sleep, stress management, and social connections—all of which are important components of a brain-healthy lifestyle. We'll also look into the potential benefits and risks of supplements and nootropics, which are tools that some people take to improve their cognitive function.

Furthermore, this book will empower you to set personal brain health objectives, inspire you to adopt a continual improvement mindset and present practical strategies for cultivating a brain-healthy lifestyle.

The endeavor to develop the brain is about more than just improving cognitive ability; it is also about improving one's quality of life. A healthier, more vibrant brain can contribute to increased creativity, emotional well-being, improved problem-solving abilities, and a stronger connection with our surroundings.

As you embark on this trip, keep in mind that developing your brain is a lifelong journey, not a destination. Each chapter will serve as a stepping stone, leading you to a deeper understanding of your brain and offering specific strategies to maximize its potential.

So, let us begin on this thrilling journey into the human brain and discover the secrets of a sharper, healthier, and more brilliant mind together.

First Chapter

The Human Brain

The human brain is the most sophisticated mechanism and important organ in the body. It is in charge of our ideas, emotions, memories, and behaviors and serves as the command center for all physical activities. This three-pound organ is home to 86 billion neurons that communicate via trillions of synapses. Everything from basic survival functions like breathing and heart rate to advanced cognitive activities like problem-solving and creativity is controlled by it.

Recognizing the importance of the brain entails acknowledging its role in defining our identity and experiences. It is the origin of awareness, allowing us to observe and interact with our surroundings. Our existence as we know it would cease to exist if our brains were not healthy and functional.

The Plasticity of the Brain:

Neuroplasticity, also known as brain plasticity, is the brain's extraordinary ability to adapt and evolve throughout our lives. It's a fundamental idea in comprehending the brain's miracle. While it was originally thought that the structure and capacities of the brain were fixed in maturity, research has demonstrated that the brain remains highly adaptable and may reorganize itself in response to learning, experience, and damage.

We can learn new skills, recover from brain damage, and adapt to changing situations thanks to neuroplasticity. It is the reason humans can learn new languages, gain competence in numerous disciplines, and regain skills following strokes or catastrophic brain injuries. Accepting the concept of neuroplasticity permits people to consistently improve their brain function through deliberate efforts.

Setting Reasonable Expectations:

Setting reasonable expectations is critical as we investigate the marvel of the brain. Although the brain is extremely adaptive and capable of growth and progress, it is not an infinite resource. Understanding the brain's boundaries and limitations is critical for creating attainable goals for brain improvement.

Setting reasonable expectations entails acknowledging that cognitive growth may necessitate time, effort, and consistency. It is not a quick fix, but rather a lifelong endeavor. Furthermore, individual variances influence how people respond to brain-enhancing treatments. What works for one individual might not work for another.

Understanding the wonder of the brain entails understanding its central role in our lives, appreciating its incredible adaptability, and establishing practical and attainable goals for brain enhancement. This core understanding lays the groundwork for investigating numerous strategies and procedures for improving brain health and cognitive performance.

Second Chapter

Brain Health Nutrition

Our diet has a significant impact on our cognitive function and mental well-being. A well-balanced diet includes vitamins, minerals, antioxidants, and macronutrients such as carbohydrates, lipids, and proteins, all of which enhance brain function. Here's a closer look at how nutrition affects cognition:

Nutrient-Rich Foods: Eating nutrient-rich foods like leafy greens, berries, fatty fish (like salmon), nuts, and whole grains can supply essential vitamins and minerals for brain function. Omega-3 fatty acids found in fish, for example, are known to boost cognitive function, whereas antioxidants found in berries assist protect brain cells from oxidative stress.

Blood Sugar Control: The brain requires a consistent supply of glucose to function. Low glycemic index foods, such as whole grains and complex carbs, assist regulate blood sugar levels and offer a steady supply of energy to the brain. This is critical for keeping focus and avoiding mood swings.

The Gut-Brain Connection: New study indicates a strong link between the gut and the brain. A healthy gut microbiota, which is regulated by dietary choices, can have an impact on cognitive function, mood, and even memory. Consuming probiotic-rich foods such as yogurt and fiber-rich fruits and vegetables can help enhance intestinal health.

The Brain-Gut Connection

The gut-brain link is an intriguing and relatively new finding in neuroscience. It refers to the two-way communication that occurs between the stomach to the brain. a sophisticated neural network in the gut called the enteric nervous system (ENS), and numerous signaling pathways promote this link.

The Effect of the Microbiome on the Brain

The gut microbiome, which is made up of billions of microorganisms, is crucial in this interaction. It generates neurotransmitters such as serotonin and communicates with the brain via the vagus nerve. A diversified and well-balanced microbiota can improve mood, cognition, and overall brain function.

Probiotics and Prebiotics: What Are They?

Probiotics are healthy bacteria that can be obtained through fermented foods or supplements. They can support the preservation of a balanced gut microbiome. Prebiotics, on the other hand, are non-digestible fibers that provide nourishment to these helpful bacteria. A diet rich in prebiotics and probiotics can aid in the promotion of a healthy gut flora.

Maintaining Gut Health

In order to keep the gut-brain connection strong, it is essential to maintain intestinal health. This entails reducing your use of processed foods, sugar, and synthetic additives, all of which have the potential to be harmful to your microbiota. Instead, concentrate on a diet rich in fiber, fermented foods, and a wide variety of fruits and vegetables.

Understanding the gut-brain connection highlights the significance of not only what we eat but also how it affects our entire health. A healthy stomach can improve your mood, lower inflammation, and boost your cognitive performance.

The book "Nutrition for Brain Health" emphasizes the importance of nutrition in cognitive function and brain health. It emphasizes the importance of eating nutrient-rich foods, controlling blood sugar levels, and maintaining a healthy gut in order to enhance brain function and overall well-being.

Physical Activity and Brain Power

Physical activity has been shown to significantly improve brain health and cognitive performance. One of its most remarkable properties is its capacity to induce neurogenesis, or the formation of new neurons in the brain. Here's an in-depth examination into the relationship between exercise and neurogenesis:

Aerobic vs. strength Training: Both aerobic exercise (such as running, swimming, or brisk walking) and strength training (such as weightlifting or bodyweight exercises) are beneficial to brain health. Aerobic exercise improves blood flow and oxygen delivery to the brain, whereas resistance training promotes the release of neurogenesis-stimulating growth factors.

Choosing the Right Exercise program: It is critical to select an exercise program that you enjoy and can stick to in the long run. Consistency is essential. Even moderate-intensity exercise for as little as 30 minutes each day can improve brain health.

Mindfulness and Yoga for Mental Clarity

Yoga and mindfulness meditation, in addition to regular physical workouts, help with mental clarity and brain power:

Stress Reduction: Relaxation, deep breathing, and stress reduction are all emphasized in yoga and mindfulness practices. Stress reduction can protect the brain from the negative effects of chronic stress and improve cognitive performance.

Yoga for Improved Concentration: Yoga combines physical postures, breathing exercises, and meditation. These ingredients can improve focus and concentration, allowing you to tackle cognitive activities with more clarity.

Mindfulness Meditation: Mindfulness meditation entails paying attention to the present moment without judgment. Meditation practice on a regular basis can increase attention, memory, and overall cognitive function.

Extra Brain-Boosting Exercises

i. **Brain Training Games:** Sudoku, crossword puzzles, and brain-training apps (such as Lumosity and Peak) test your cognitive talents. They improve problem-solving abilities, memory, and logical reasoning.

ii. **Playing an Instrument:** Learning to play an instrument, such as the piano, guitar, or violin, simultaneously engages a number of different brain regions. Memory, coordination, and creative thinking are all enhanced.

iii. **Dance**: Ballroom, hip-hop, and salsa dancing all mix physical exercise with sophisticated movement patterns and synchronization. It improves mood, cognition, and social interaction.

iv. **Tai Chi:** Tai Chi is a leisurely and graceful type of exercise that combines gentle motions and deep breathing. It improves balance, flexibility, and cognition. Tai Chi can be especially good for seniors.

v. **Juggling**: Juggling is a fascinating and difficult activity that involves hand-eye coordination and focus. Juggling can excite the brain and enhance coordination.

vi. **Mental Math:** Use mental math exercises to test your arithmetic abilities and develop your mental agility. Begin with simple calculations and work your way up in complexity.

Including a variety of physical exercises and brain-boosting activities in your daily routine can help you reap the most benefits for your brain health. Remember that consistency and enjoyment are important aspects in establishing a long-term fitness plan that promotes cognitive function and brain capacity.

Fourth Chapter

Cognitive Training and Mental Stimulation

Engaging in activities that challenge and excite various cognitive functions, such as memory, problem-solving, and creativity, constitutes mental stimulation. Here's how mental stimulation benefits the brain in more detail:

Crossword Puzzles and Brain activities: Crossword puzzles, Sudoku, and brain-training activities such as chess or memory games can help to improve memory and analytical thinking. These activities stimulate the brain's ability to connect and think critically.

Acquiring New abilities: Acquiring new abilities, such as learning a foreign language or playing a musical instrument, increases brain plasticity. It stimulates brain areas involved in memory, multitasking, and linguistic abilities.

Reading and Critical Thinking: Regular reading, particularly of complex and difficult material, fosters a deeper comprehension of concepts and promotes critical thinking. It increases vocabulary and improves comprehension.

Brain Training and Mindfulness

While mindfulness techniques are primarily concerned with mental health, they also benefit cognitive training and brain health:

i. **Mindful Breathing:** Deep breathing exercises, which are an essential component of mindfulness, can reduce stress and anxiety, enhance relaxation, and increase attention span. This is very useful for people who want to improve their concentration.

ii. **Mindful Observation:** Mindfulness promotes acute awareness of one's thoughts, feelings, and environment. This increased awareness can result in improved self-regulation and emotional intelligence, both of which are important components of cognitive performance.

iii. **Mindful Living:** Practicing mindfulness in daily life fosters a state of present and awareness. This can contribute to enhanced decision-making, resilience, and overall cognitive well-being.

Cognitive Training with Structure

Structured cognitive training consists of exercises and activities that are meant to improve certain cognitive functions. Beyond broad mental stimulation, this technique focuses on deliberate practice to increase cognitive function:

i. **Memory Exercises:** Memory exercises can assist people of all ages improve their recall abilities. Memory techniques such as mnemonic devices, memory games, and spaced repetition can help to improve memory.

ii. **Focus and Attention Training:** Attention is a crucial cognitive function. Meditation or specific attention-focused games are examples of training exercises that help increase concentration and eliminate distractions.

iii. **Problem-Solving and Critical Thinking:** Problem-solving games, logical puzzles, and strategy games such as chess can help improve problem-solving and critical thinking skills.

iv. **Processing Speed:** Some cognitive training regimens aim to increase the brain's processing speed. These workouts force the brain to respond to stimuli more quickly, which may improve reaction time and decision-making.

Integrating mental stimulation, mindfulness techniques, and structured cognitive training into your everyday routine can assist maximize brain health and cognitive function. The idea is to keep your brain busy and adaptive throughout your life, whether you want to engage in hard puzzles, acquire a new skill, practice mindfulness, or follow a systematic cognitive training program.

Fifth Chapter

Sleep Quality for Cognitive Enhancement

Sleep is necessary for general brain health and cognitive performance. It performs several critical roles that promote brain health:

Memory Consolidation: The brain consolidates memories during deep sleep stages, sorting and storing information obtained throughout the day. This procedure is critical for acquiring and retaining new information.

Emotional Regulation: Adequate sleep aids in emotion regulation and mood stability. It alleviates irritation, anxiety, and stress, all of which have an affect on cognitive performance.

Neuroplasticity: Sleep is important for brain plasticity because it allows the brain to adapt and restructure itself. This is critical for learning new knowledge and adapting to new situations.

Sleep Patterns: Understanding the sleep cycle is essential for improving sleep quality:

Sleep Stages: Sleep is divided into stages, including REM (rapid eye movement) and non-REM. Each stage has a distinct purpose, such as deep restorative sleep in the non-REM stages and dreaming and memory consolidation in the REM stages.

Sleep Cycle Length: The sleep cycle lasts around 90 minutes and is repeated throughout the night. It's critical to get multiple full sleep cycles in order to wake up feeling refreshed.

Sleep Deprivation's Effects: Chronic sleep loss has been shown to have negative consequences on cognitive performance and general health:

Cognitive Impairment: Sleep deprivation can result in decreased attention, diminished memory, decreased problem-solving ability, and slower reaction times.

Emotional Disturbance: Sleep deprivation frequently causes mood changes, irritability, and elevated stress levels.

Consequences for Physical Health: Lack of sleep over a long period of time has been associated with an increased risk of obesity, diabetes, and cardiovascular disease.

Making Your Bedroom Sleep-Friendly:

The quality of your sleep may be significantly impacted by creating the optimum sleeping environment:

Invest in a comfy mattress and pillows that suit your preferences. Maintain a pleasant temperature in your bedroom.

Eliminate Noise and Light: Use blackout curtains to block off outdoor light, and white noise machines or earplugs to eliminate distracting sounds.

Techniques to Enhance Sleep Quality:

Good Sleep Hygiene Advice: You can develop healthy sleeping habits by using proper sleep hygiene:

Keep a Regular Sleep Schedule: Attempt to go to bed and wake up at the same times every day, including on the weekends.

Limit Screen Time: Limit your exposure to screens (phones, tablets, laptops, and televisions) before bedtime because the blue light emitted can interrupt your sleep.

Avoid Heavy Meals and Caffeine Before Bed: Eat substantial meals and avoid caffeine several hours before bedtime to give your body time to digest and unwind.

Relaxation activities: The following relaxation activities might help calm the mind and prepare it for rest:

Deep Breathing: Deep breathing techniques can help you relax your body and lessen stress.

Progressive Muscle Relaxation: To relieve physical tension, tense and then release each muscle group in your body.

Managing Sleep Disorders: Seek professional help if you feel you have a sleep condition, such as insomnia or sleep apnea. Sleep disorders can have a substantial impact on cognitive performance and overall health, but they are frequently curable with the appropriate interventions.

You'll sleep better by incorporating these concepts and techniques into your daily routine, improve your cognitive performance, and improve your general brain health. Prioritizing excellent sleep is a critical step toward improving cognitive performance and overall well-being.

Stress Reduction and Emotional Well-Being

"Stress Management and Emotional Well-being," which covers the brain's response to stress, the HPA axis, and the effects of chronic stress before moving on to stress reduction measures.

The Stress Response of the Brain:

Stress is a natural reaction to perceived threats or difficulties, and the brain is central to this response. Understanding how the brain reacts to stress is critical for effective stress management:

The Hypothalamus-Pituitary-Adrenal (HPA) Axis: The Hypothalamus-Pituitary-Adrenal (HPA) axis is an important aspect of the stress response system. When the hypothalamus detects stress, it secretes corticotropin-releasing hormone (CRH), which triggers the pituitary gland to secrete adrenocorticotropic hormone (ACTH). In turn, ACTH causes the adrenal glands to release stress hormones including cortisol and adrenaline.

Persistent Stress Effects: While the stress response is adaptive in the short term, persistent stress can be harmful to the brain and overall health. Prolonged stress hormone elevation can cause anxiety, depression, decreased memory and cognitive function, and an increased risk of several health disorders, including cardiovascular disease.

Stress Reduction Techniques:

In order to properly manage stress and enhance emotional well-being, the following stress reduction techniques must be used:

Deep breathing techniques, such as diaphragmatic breathing or the 4-7-8 technique, help stimulate the relaxation response in the body. These exercises aid in the reduction of stress hormones, the reduction of blood pressure, and the promotion of a sense of calm.

Meditation and Mindfulness: Mindfulness practices entail paying nonjudgmental attention to the present moment. Meditation approaches that promote relaxation, emotional control, and enhanced attention, such as mindfulness meditation or loving-kindness meditation, can help relieve stress.

Stress-Relieving Activities: Stress-relieving activities such as physical exercise, hobbies, and time spent in nature can help lower stress. Endorphins, which are natural mood boosters, are released during exercise, and outdoor activities can relieve stress and increase mood.

Other stress management measures could include:

Time Management: To avoid feeling overwhelmed, prioritize work, set reasonable goals, and divide projects into manageable steps.

Social Support: Creating and maintaining a solid support network can provide emotional support during times of stress. Stress can be managed by talking to friends, family, or a therapist.

Choices for a Healthy Lifestyle: A balanced diet, regular exercise, and adequate rest are all examples of healthy lifestyle choices that can assist the body in coping with stress.

Relaxation Techniques: Techniques like progressive muscle relaxation, biofeedback, and aromatherapy can help you relax and reduce stress.

Incorporating these stress-reduction tactics into your daily routine will help you control your brain's stress response, lessen the effects of chronic stress, and improve your overall emotional well-being. You can improve cognitive performance and retain a positive attitude on life by minimizing stress.

<u>Seventh Chapter</u>

Social Relationships and Brain Health

Humans are social organisms by nature, and our brains have evolved to flourish in social settings. According to the social brain idea, our ability to interact with people and develop complex social relationships has played an important part in the evolution of our species. This idea emphasizes the importance of social relationships in human existence, as well as their substantial impact on brain health.

Mirror Neurons: Mirror neurons are specialized brain cells that fire when we do an action as well as when we witness someone else performing the same action. They are supposed to help us understand and empathize with others, which improves our ability to learn from others and develop societies.

Emotional Contagion: Emotional responses in the brain are triggered by social interactions. We can "catch" other people's emotions when we engage with them, whether they are happy, sad, or stressed. This emotional contagion emphasizes how interrelated our emotional experiences are.

The Effects of Social Exclusion:

Social isolation and loneliness, on the other hand, can have a negative impact on brain health and overall well-being. Long-term social isolation can result in:

Cognitive Decline: Research has connected social isolation to cognitive decline as well as an increased risk of neurodegenerative disorders such as Alzheimer's.

Loneliness: Loneliness has been linked to an increased risk of sadness, anxiety, and other mental health conditions. Emotional anguish can be exacerbated by a lack of social relationships.

Physical Health Implications: Social isolation can have an influence on physical health by increasing inflammation, weakening immunological function, and increasing the risk of chronic diseases.

Making Meaningful Connections:

Building and maintaining meaningful social relationships is an important element of brain and emotional wellness. Here are some ideas for cultivating such relationships:

Active Listening: The foundation of any healthy relationship is effective communication. Listen to others actively, convey empathy, and validate their feelings and experiences.

Quality Time: Make time to cultivate relationships. Spend time with loved ones, hold meaningful conversations, and create shared experiences.

Seek out and establish helpful relationships in which you may both provide and receive emotional support. Individual ties are strengthened by mutual assistance.

Healthy limits: Keep healthy limits in your relationships, making sure they are balanced and supportive of your well-being. Boundaries aid in the prevention of emotional weariness and the preservation of personal space.

Nutrient-Rich Diet

Your brain is a high-performance organ that is continuously working to analyze information, regulate physical functions, and guide your thoughts and activities. It requires sufficient nutrition to work at its best. Just like a well-tuned engine requires high-quality gasoline to function properly, your brain requires a well-balanced and nutrient-rich diet to thrive.

Nutritional Needs of the Brain:

Your brain is a voracious organ, consuming roughly 20% of your daily energy intake. It requires a regular supply of vital nutrients to function properly. A brain-boosting diet should include the following ingredients:

Omega-3 Fatty Acids: Found in fatty fish such as salmon, walnuts, and flaxseeds, these healthful fats are essential for brain construction and function. They promote cell membrane development, increase communication between brain cells, and may lessen the risk of cognitive decline.

Antioxidants: Antioxidant-rich foods like berries, dark chocolate, and colorful veggies protect the brain against oxidative stress and inflammation. As a result, memory and cognitive function may improve.

Vitamins and minerals: B-vitamins (especially B6, B9, and B12), vitamin D, and minerals like zinc and magnesium all play important roles in cognitive performance, mood control, and brain growth.

Protein: Amino acids derived from protein sources such as lean meat, chicken, fish, beans, and tofu are the building blocks of neurotransmitters, which are chemical messengers in the brain that allow brain cells to communicate with one another.

Whole grains, legumes, and vegetables provide a consistent supply of glucose, the brain's principal source of energy. Complex carbs gradually release glucose, promoting consistent energy levels and cognitive performance.

The Brain-Gut Connection:

The intricate connection that exists between the gut and the brain has been clarified by recent investigations. The billions of bacteria that reside in your digestive tract and make up your gut microbiome can affect how well your brain functions. A diet rich in fiber and fermented foods (like kimchi and yogurt) may aid in maintaining a healthy gut flora, which may enhance mood, cognition, and general brain function.

It's Important to Stay Hydrated:

Staying hydrated is essential for brain health. Mild dehydration can have a negative impact on cognitive function, focus, and mood. Drink plenty of water throughout the day, and think about eating hydrating foods like watermelon, cucumber, and herbal teas.

Foods that Improve Memory:

Here are some things to include in your diet to help with brain health:

- Fatty Fish: Omega-3 fatty acids are abundant in salmon, mackerel, and sardines.
- Leafy Greens: Spinach, kale, and Swiss chard are high in antioxidants and vitamins.
- Berries: Antioxidants abound in blueberries, strawberries, and blackberries.
- Nuts and Seeds: Healthy fats can be found in walnuts, almonds, flaxseeds, and chia seeds.
- Whole Grains: Complex carbs can be found in oats, quinoa, and brown rice.
- Lean Proteins: Chicken, turkey, lean beef, and tofu are all good sources of vital amino acids.
- Colorful Vegetables: Bell peppers, carrots, and sweet potatoes are high in antioxidants and vitamins.

Balance and moderation:

While including brain-boosting nutrients in your diet is vital, so is maintaining balance and moderation. Avoid eating too many processed meals, sugary snacks, and trans fats, which can have a negative impact on brain function.

A brain-boosting diet is a long-term investment in your cognitive health and overall well-being, not a short fix. You can improve memory, focus, mood, and even minimize the risk of age-related cognitive decline by supporting your brain with a range of nutrient-rich meals. Make intelligent food purchases and prioritize a diet that nourishes not only your body but also your wonderful, high-performing brain.

Social Activities that Improve the Brain

Group Learning and Hobbies: Participating in group learning and hobbies can provide cognitive stimulation while also strengthening social connections:

Study Groups, Book Clubs, and Discussion Groups: Participating in a study group, book club, or discussion group can stimulate your mind through intellectual exchanges while also developing social relationships with like-minded others.

Creative Hobbies: Engaging in creative hobbies such as painting, writing, or music in a group setting can improve cognitive capacities, spark creativity, and provide a sense of togetherness.

Volunteering is a meaningful method to give back to society while enjoying cognitive and emotional benefits:

A Sense of Purpose: Volunteering can give you a sense of purpose and fulfillment, which can improve your overall well-being and self-esteem.

Social Engagement: Volunteering frequently entails teamwork and engagement with others, which helps to improve social relationships and maybe form new friendships.

Skill Development: Depending on the volunteer activity, you can learn new skills and get new knowledge, which promotes cognitive growth.

Family and friendships are the foundation of societies and provide several brain-boosting benefits:

Emotional Support: During difficult times, trusted friends and family provide emotional support, decreasing stress and boosting emotional well-being.

Shared Memories and Experiences: Sharing experiences and memories with loved ones weaves a rich tapestry of life, increasing cognitive function by stimulating memory recall and establishing emotional relationships.

Brain Health in Aging: In midlife and beyond, strong social relationships are connected with greater cognitive health and a lower risk of cognitive decline and dementia.

Social relationships are inextricably linked to brain health and emotional well-being. Our brains are hardwired to thrive in social settings, where we can benefit from meaningful interactions, emotional support, and cognitive stimulation. Contrarily, social isolation may be detrimental to one's physical and mental health. Individuals can improve their cognitive function, emotional resilience, and general quality of life by actively building social connections and engaging in brain-boosting social activities. Prioritizing social interactions is critical to sustaining a healthy and vibrant brain throughout life.

<u>**Eight Chapter**</u>

Nootropics and Brain Enhancement Supplements

Supplements can help promote cognitive performance and brain health, but they are not a replacement for a healthy lifestyle. The following supplements have been examined for their possible cognitive benefits:

- Omega-3 Fatty Acids: Omega-3 fatty acids, specifically EPA (eicosapentaenoic acid) and DHA (docosahexaenoic acid) found in fatty fish such as salmon and mackerel, have been linked to better cognitive performance. They are thought to benefit brain health by lowering inflammation, encouraging brain cell membrane development, and increasing synaptic plasticity.

- Vitamin D: Vitamin D, also known as the "sunshine vitamin," is essential for many biological activities, including brain health. Low vitamin D levels have been related to cognitive decline as well as an increased risk of neurodegenerative disorders. Ensuring appropriate vitamin D consumption, whether from sunlight or pills, may aid cognitive performance.

- Herbal Supplements: The cognitive benefits of several herbal supplements have been investigated. Ginkgo biloba, which may boost blood flow to the brain and memory, and ginseng, which has been linked to improved cognitive ability, are two examples.

Investigating Nootropics

Nootropics, sometimes known as "smart drugs" or cognitive enhancers, are compounds that some people take to improve their cognitive performance. There are numerous nootropics, each with its unique set of mechanisms and potential benefits:

Racetams: Racetams are a type of synthetic nootropic that includes piracetam and aniracetam. They are said to help with memory, learning, and cognitive function.

Cholinergics: Precursors of the neurotransmitter acetylcholine, such as choline and alpha-GPC. They are believed to aid memory and learning.

Adaptogens: Adaptogenic herbs such as rhodiola rosea and ashwagandha may aid in stress adaptation and increase cognitive resilience.

Stimulants: Modafinil and coffee, for example, are stimulants that can boost alertness and focus.

Potential Advantages and Drawbacks of Nootropics:

Nootropics have gained popularity due to their possible cognitive-enhancing effects, but it is critical to weigh both the advantages and disadvantages:

Potential Advantages:

Nootropics have the potential to increase memory, concentration, and mental clarity. Some users claim to have more creativity and motivation. However, the effects can vary greatly between individuals.

Potential Risks:

The long-term safety and efficacy of several nootropics remain unknown. Some nootropics may cause negative effects, interact with other drugs, or be abused. Before utilizing them, it is critical to consult with a healthcare expert.

Responsible Use:

If you decide to experiment with nootropics, it is critical that you do it responsibly:

- **Consult a Healthcare Professional:** Before beginning any nootropic program, evaluate potential hazards and benefits with a healthcare provider, especially if you have underlying health concerns or are taking other drugs.

- **Research and dose:** Research the exact nootropic you intend to use thoroughly, including dose recommendations. Begin with the lowest effective dose and track your progress.

- **Quality and Purity**: To reduce the possibility of contaminants or impurities, purchase high-quality, respected items.

- **Keep an eye on the effects**: Pay attention to how the nootropic impacts you. If you encounter any side effects or discomfort, stop using the product and consult a healthcare expert.

Finally, vitamins and nootropics can be thought of as instruments for enhancing cognitive performance and brain health. While some supplements, such as omega-3 fatty acids and vitamin D, have well-documented advantages, nootropics are a broad group of compounds with varying degrees of scientific backing. When considering the usage of supplements and nootropics for cognitive development, it is critical to make informed decisions and speak with a healthcare practitioner. Furthermore, a comprehensive approach to brain health must be prioritized, which includes a healthy lifestyle, nutrition, exercise, and social interactions.

The Journey to a Better Brain

The importance of setting personal objectives, striving for continual development, and adopting a brain-healthy lifestyle as critical components of the journey to improving cognitive function and general brain health.

Setting Personal Goals: Improving your brain health is a very personalized journey, and the first step is to create clear, attainable goals. Personalized goals enable you to define what a "better brain" means to you and sketch out a path to get there. Here's how to go about making goals:

Establish Priorities: Consider which areas of brain health and cognitive function are most important to you. Is it for memory enhancement, stress reduction, creative enhancement, or something else?

Set Specific and Measurable Goals: Your objectives should be specific, measurable, and time-bound. Instead of a general objective like "improve memory," set a specific target like "increase memory recall by 20% within six months."

Divide Goals Into Actionable actions: Divide larger goals into smaller, more achievable actions. This makes them less intimidating and allows you to track your progress.

Stay Motivated: Review your goals on a regular basis and appreciate your accomplishments along the way. Positive reinforcement can aid with motivational retention.

Continuous Improvement: Improving brain health is a continuous process, not a one-time effort. It necessitates a dedication to constant improvement and learning. Here are some ideas for embracing constant growth:

Lifelong Learning: Keep your mind active by learning new abilities, such as a new language, musical instrument, or hobby. Continuous learning both challenges and encourages neuroplasticity in the brain.

Be Curious: Develop an interest in the world around you. Pose questions, seek solutions, and investigate new ideas. Curiosity is a powerful motivator for mental engagement.

Mindful Practice: Make mindfulness a part of your daily routine. Practice being present, paying attention to your thoughts and emotions, and effectively handling stress.

Adapt and Adjust: Be adaptable and open to new experiences. If a specific brain-boosting strategy isn't functioning as planned, don't be afraid to change your approach and try different methods.

Adopting a Brain-Healthy Lifestyle: Adopting a brain-healthy lifestyle that incorporates multiple facets of well-being is critical to supporting your journey to a better brain:

Nutrition: Eat a well-balanced diet that is high in brain-boosting nutrients such as omega-3 fatty acids, antioxidants, and vitamins. Stay hydrated and limit your intake of processed meals and sugars.

Physical Activity: Include frequent physical activity in your regimen. Aerobic exercise, strength training, and activities such as yoga all help to improve brain health.

Quality Sleep: Make sleep a priority and develop healthy sleeping habits. A regular sleep schedule, a pleasant sleeping environment, and stress-reduction practices can all help to improve sleep quality.

Stress Reduction: Use stress-reduction practices like mindfulness, meditation, and relaxation exercises. To protect your brain from the negative consequences of persistent stress, learn how to manage stress efficiently.

• Social Relationships: Develop meaningful relationships and social connections. Engage with friends and loved ones on a regular basis to promote emotional well-being.

• Use of Supplements and Nootropics with Caution: If you choose to use supplements or nootropics, do so with caution, under the supervision of a healthcare expert, and as part of a whole brain-healthy lifestyle.

Finally, the quest for a better brain is a lifelong undertaking based on personal goals, constant growth, and the adoption of a brain-healthy lifestyle. You may improve cognitive performance and enjoy the benefits of a healthy and vibrant brain throughout your life by setting clear goals, staying committed to progress, and nurturing your brain through nutrition, exercise, sleep, stress management, and social relationships. Keep in mind that every step you take toward a healthy brain improves your entire well-being and quality of life.